The Employment and Distributional Effects of Mandated Benefits

June E. O'Neill and Dave M. O'Neill

The AEI Press

Publisher for the American Enterprise Institute

WASHINGTON, D.C.

1994

To order call toll free 1-800-462-6420 or 1-717-794-3800. For all other inquiries please contact the AEI Press, 1150 Seventeenth Street, N.W., Washington, D.C. 20036 or call 1-800-862-5801.

ISBN 978-0-8447-7021-5

ISBN 0-8447-7021-3

THE AEI PRESS
Publisher for the American Enterprise Institute
1150 17th Street, N.W., Washington, D.C. 20036

Contents

In his State of the Union Address on January 26, 1994, President Clinton made it clear that the major goal of his health plan is to guarantee universal health insurance coverage for all Americans. To achieve this goal, the Clinton plan relies primarily on a mandate requiring all employers to pay up to 80 percent of the cost of health insurance premiums for their workers.[1] About 66 million wage-and-salary workers currently receive insurance benefits from their employers. Under the Clinton plan, other employers who do not now provide coverage would be required to cover an additional 45 million workers—even though all but 18 million of these workers are already covered through other means, such as a spouse's employer-based policy (table 1). Those who have no working family member eligible for the plan face an individual mandate requiring that they enroll in the plan and pay the full premium, with subsidies provided for low-income individuals.

An employer mandate has considerable political appeal, particularly to a government facing large budget deficits. It appears to finance health insurance for the vast majority of Americans, not by raising their taxes but by sending the "bill" to employers. A main selling point of the Clinton administration has been that companies not now providing insurance to their workers are getting "what amounts to a free ride."[2] But a near consensus prevails among economists who study these matters that employers ultimately pass most of the costs of health benefits to workers, who pay the bill through lower wages, and where wage rollbacks are infeasible, through reductions in employment. Thus, firms that provide health benefits to their workers are not at any competitive disadvantage relative to those that do not provide coverage. In other words, there is no such thing as a "free ride."

This study draws on material in June E. O'Neill and Dave M. O'Neill, *The Impact of a Health Insurance Mandate on Labor Costs and Employment: Empirical Evidence* (Employment Policies Institute, September 1993); and June E. O'Neill and Dave M. O'Neill, *Effects of the Employer Mandate in the Clinton Health Plan* (Employment Policies Institute and Center for the Study of Business and Government, February 1994). The authors acknowledge the expert programming assistance of Wenhui Li.

1

TABLE 1
CURRENT HEALTH INSURANCE STATUS OF WAGE AND SALARY WORKERS
SUBJECT TO THE CLINTON MANDATE

	Number of Workers (millions)	Percent of Category	Percent of Total
Workers not insured by own employer			
Covered by spouse's employer	15.2	33.7	13.7
Covered by other sources	11.7	25.9	10.5
No insurance from any source	18.3	40.4	16.5
Total	45.1	100.0	40.6
Workers insured by own employer			
Plan covers self only	28.7	43.5	25.8
Plan covers family	37.3	56.5	33.6
Total	66.0	100.0	59.4
All workers subject to mandate	111.1		100.0

SOURCE: Tabulated from U.S. Bureau of the Census, *Current Population Survey (CPS) March 1993*, public use file. All wage-and-salary workers are subject to the mandate unless they worked less than ten hours a week, were under age eighteen, or were full-time students under the age of twenty-four. The table includes workers meeting these terms who had work experience during 1992.

Effects of the Clinton Mandate

The impact of an employer mandate is a matter of concern because it falls largely on uninsured workers, and these workers primarily earn low wages: close to half earn less than $6.50 an hour. In consequence, the mandated premium would impose a particularly sharp increase in the compensation an employer must pay to these workers—an estimated 16 percent increase for the average uninsured worker, rising to 25 percent in very low-wage industries such as "eating and drinking." Yet the ability of employers to pass such large compensation increases on to their low-wage employees in the form of reduced pay is extremely limited. Many of these workers are at or close to the minimum wage, and the firm cannot legally lower their wage to absorb the higher health costs. As a result, some workers will lose their jobs as firms seek to replace low-skill workers in the uncovered sector with high-skill workers or with automated equipment; or firms find that it has become too costly to remain in the affected industries.

The Clinton administration was evidently aware of this problem and in drafting its plan has tried to soften the negative effects of the mandate by providing subsidies to small firms with low-wage workers. But while these subsidies would significantly diminish the potential job loss, they do not eliminate it. Our estimates suggest that about 2.1 million workers would lose their jobs if the Clinton mandate were implemented without any subsidies. Yet even with the subsidies, significant job losses in the range of 500,000 to 900,000 would still occur. Because a substantial part of the costs is shifted to workers, wages of formerly uninsured workers would also decline—on average, by about 6 percent, even after taking account of the subsidies.

Although the proposed premium subsidies to employers reduce the potential job loss in the uncovered sector, they also create a new set of problems. First, they will necessitate large annual increases in federal expenditures: an estimated $40 billion if the plan had been in effect in 1993. In addition, the peculiar incentives generated by the subsidies are likely to lead to losses in economic productivity as firms reorganize their work forces to lower their health insurance costs.

The effects of the Clinton mandate are bound to be complex because the plan imposes different combinations of cost increases and cost reductions on the covered and uncovered sectors of the labor force. The effects would also differ by industry and by personal characteristics such as marital and family status: two-earner couples, for example, would fare particularly badly. This study examines the effects of the mandate on wage-and-salary workers and on the efficiency of resource allocation in the economy. Estimates are provided on the effect of the mandate on employment, wages, and federal expenditures.

It is important to recognize that a wide margin of uncertainty surrounds any estimates of the effects of the Clinton plan. Political events that can only be matters for speculation can greatly affect the outcome. Premium subsidies to firms, for example, might be substantially scaled back by Congress if they should prove to be a budget buster. But such efforts to reduce observable budget expenditures will certainly increase the extent of employment cutbacks and wage reductions. No one can predict the ultimate expenditures or other aspects of the system when cost controllers in government and in the alliances that manage the plan are pitted against a public that may well press its representatives for increasingly generous benefits.

Economic factors that cannot be reliably predicted will also have significant effects on the mandate. If the trend of the past fifteen years is maintained, the labor market for low-skill workers will continue to

3

decline with downward pressure on real wages. In this case, the disemployment effects of the mandate would be more severe than we have estimated. But if the situation should reverse and wages for those at the bottom should begin to rise, the disemployment effects of the mandate would be reduced. To limit the enormous potential for error in projecting the state of the economy in 1998, when the Clinton plan is to be operational in all states, we have made all our estimates as though the plan had been in effect in calendar year 1993.

Key Assumptions of the Estimates

The estimates presented are necessarily influenced by certain key assumptions. These assumptions cover (1) the likely cost of premiums under the plan; (2) the extent to which wages can be reduced to pay for the premiums; and (3) the extent to which labor demand responds to the unabsorbed wage cost increase (the so-called elasticity of labor demand).

Premiums. The premium cost of the basic plan clearly drives its economic impacts by influencing the rise in labor costs associated with the mandate and, therefore, the costs of the employer and employee subsidies and the expected employment and wage effects. The administration's estimates of premium costs in 1994 are given in appendix 2 of the proposed Health Security Act. Several outside experts have concluded that the administration's assumptions of premium prices are unrealistically low, given the relatively high levels of benefits promised in the Health Security Act. Excluding the dental component (the Clinton plan does not cover adult dental care until 2000), Hewitt Associates ranked the Clinton plan's package of medical benefits as somewhat above average when compared with that of the typical large private employer.[3]

Table 2 compares the Hewitt actuaries' pricing of the cost for the standard Clinton plan with that of the administration. The Clinton plan provides for a four-tier price structure—three categories of families and single individuals—rather than the more common two-tier structure that distinguishes only families and individuals. As shown, the Hewitt estimates exceed the administration estimates by 26 percent for individuals and couples with no children and by 59 percent for a couple with children. Thus, in addition to differences in the premium prices, the actuarial model used by Hewitt Associates produces a different pricing structure from that of the administration.

Several factors may explain why Hewitt's (and others') estimates of premium prices are higher than the administration's. One source of difference is likely to arise from assumptions about use of medical services after the plan is implemented. For insurance purposes, the Clinton plan pools the Medicaid and the uninsured populations with the working population that is already insured and requires that health care charges be

TABLE 2
ESTIMATED ANNUAL PREMIUM COST FOR HEALTH PLAN BENEFITS
IF PROVIDED IN 1993,
BASED ON ALTERNATIVE SOURCES
(dollars)

Combined Employer and Employee Share

Family type	Administration	HIAA	Hewitt Associates	Foster Higgins
Single person	1,768	2,110	2,200	2,250
Two adults	3,536	4,425	4,460	4,510
One adult and children	3,562	4,200	4,200	5,350
Two adults and children	3,989	6,300	6,300	5,970

Employer Share

Family type	Administration	HIAA	Hewitt Associates	Foster Higgins
Single person	1,414	1,688	1,760	1,800
Two adults	1,944	2,432	2,452	2,480
One adult and children	2,268	2,674	2,694	3,414
Two adults and children	2,268	3,582	3,582	3,414

NOTE: Administration estimates for the four family tiers are given in appendix 2 of the proposed Health Security Act for 1994. They were reduced by 8.5 percent to approximate 1993 levels. Hewitt Associates estimates for the four tiers were given in testimony before the U.S. Subcommittee on Health and the Environment, Committee on Energy and Commerce, November 22, 1993 (Hewitt 1994 estimates were scaled back to 1993 levels). Premium data from the annual survey of the Health Insurance Association of America (HIAA) for 1991 were projected to 1993. (Premiums for a two-tier structure—individual and family average only—were converted into a four-tier structure.) Foster Higgins 1993 estimates for a two-tier structure were also converted into four tiers.

community rated rather than experience rated.[4] Under community rating, all individuals in a community pay the same rate regardless of their expected use of medical care. Hewitt predicts that the inclusion of the Medicaid and uninsured groups will raise per person insurance costs by 6 percent, because the new groups are estimated to be significantly more costly to insure.

A second source of differences in estimates derives from assumptions about the extent to which private premium costs would decline once uncompensated care costs are reduced. The administration has factored into its estimates of premiums the expectation that substantial cost savings to private insurance (a 15 percent reduction) would be realized because of an expected decline in cost shifting. By cost shifting is meant a supposed practice by which hospital charges to private insurers are increased to pay for uncompensated care (charity care plus bad debt) as well as for the unreimbursed costs of Medicare and Medicaid patients. But the actual size of the cost-shift factor embedded in private insurance premiums is a controversial matter.[5] Therefore, the size of any decline in private premiums as a result of reductions in uncompensated care generated by the Clinton plan remains highly uncertain. Hewitt estimates only a 5 percent reduction in insurance costs attributable to this factor.

A third likely reason why the administration would project lower premium costs is its frequently stated expectation that the cost and price controls specified in the plan will reduce the costs of care without diminishing its quality and accessibility. But this expectation is mainly a matter of the faith one has in the Clinton plan. An increasing number of analysts outside the administration have expressed strong reservations that cost controls could long survive in the United States and have forecast much more steeply rising health care costs as universal coverage is attained.[6]

Table 2 shows two additional estimates of current premium prices. These estimates are based on two other sources of survey information concerning the premium prices that large firms actually pay for their workers' health benefits: the annual employer survey of Foster Higgins, a benefit consulting firm, and of the Health Insurance Association of America (HIAA). Although the estimates shown were not specifically designed to estimate the cost of the Clinton plan, they provide useful information on the current status of actual employer costs. The premium prices reported in the Foster Higgins and HIAA surveys are remarkably similar to the Hewitt estimates.[7]

In our simulations of the labor market and budget impacts of the mandate, we use alternative premium prices based on the administration's premium estimates as well as those of Hewitt and Foster Higgins.

Shifting Costs to Workers. How much of the increase in employer premium costs can be shifted to workers? A key determinant of the impact of a mandate is the extent to which an employer can shift premium costs to uncovered workers. Clearly, if employers could pass all the cost increases associated with the mandated benefits onto workers by reducing their money wages, there would be no impact of a mandate on employment. Total compensation would remain the same; only the distribution of compensation between cash wages and fringe benefits would change. The ease with which employers can lower money wages to pay for fringe benefits is likely to depend on both the level of the worker's wage and the value workers place on these benefits. If workers value health benefits as much as an equivalent amount of cash compensation, then full shifting can be expected. Consequently, workers who already receive health benefits through their employers are likely to have cash wages that are lower than they otherwise would have been, reflecting a trade-off that they have implicitly chosen. Employers who provide health insurance, therefore, are not at any disadvantage relative to those who do not provide such benefits. Nor are employers who do not provide benefits exploiting their workers or earning abnormal profits.

But the cost of health benefits may not be so easily shifted to uninsured workers when these benefits are mandated. Many uninsured workers are likely to have chosen not to be insured because they value the cash income more than the benefit. Included in this category would be young healthy workers or workers who already have insurance coverage through a spouse or another source.

The potential for shifting in the sector without employer-based coverage is also limited because the majority of uninsured workers earn low wages. If the uninsured worker is paid the minimum wage, it would be illegal for the firm to reduce the wage further to pay for the mandated insurance costs. Moreover, some low-wage workers may choose to withdraw from the labor market if their wages fall any lower, particularly if they have the option to go on welfare, to work in the home, or to work in the "underground economy." The provision of health insurance to nonworkers and dependents would add to the incentive to leave legal employment covered by mandate. Still another factor limiting the ability of firms to shift costs at low-wage levels is the need to maintain compensation differentials between groups of workers to reflect seniority and skills levels.

The quantitative impacts of these factors are difficult to assess except for the minimum wage, which explicitly prevents shifting to wage levels below the minimum. It is highly likely that the extent of shifting will be greater in the long run than the short run, although the timing is difficult to predict. For these reasons, we have estimated the employment impact of the Clinton plan with a range of assumptions about the extent of shifting, assumptions we believe will approximate the existing labor market constraints.

For our "most likely" scenario, we have assumed that among the currently uninsured, close to 70 percent of the cost of the new premium would be shifted to workers through lower wages.[8] We use a graduated scale, however, ranging from 100 percent shifting for full-time workers earning $300 a week or more, to partial shifting below $300, and with no further downward shifting once the hourly wage reaches $6.50. We also provide estimates assuming the maximum possible shifting of the premium down to the legal minimum wage ($4.25 per hour), which for all unin-

7

sured workers amounts to shifting of close to 80 percent of the cost of the mandate. Under this extreme shifting assumption, the number of workers earning at or below the minimum wage would more than double as a result of the implementation of the mandate.

The Employment Response. The employment impact of the Clinton mandate depends in part on the actual increase in employer costs caused by the mandate and in part on the responsiveness of employers to this cost increase. Generally speaking, the responsiveness of employment to a change in a wage or compensation increase is referred to as the wage elasticity of labor demand. It measures the percentage decline in employment associated with a 1 percent increase in compensation. The magnitude of this employer response, or wage elasticity, is partly determined by the employer's ability to substitute other inputs (such as capital equipment) for the workers whose compensation has increased; and it is also shaped by consumer behavior. If consumers can easily shift their purchases away from the products with large mandate-induced increases in labor costs, then these firms will find it difficult to pass the cost of the mandate onto consumers by raising prices.

Direct evidence on the likely size of the total response cannot be obtained because a health insurance mandate has never been imposed. But indirect evidence based on roughly analogous situations can be brought to bear on the issue. One source of evidence is the multitude of studies on the employment effects of changes in the federal minimum wage. Increases in the minimum wage are similar to the mandate in that the firm is required by law to pay a higher cost for certain workers; and in both cases, low-wage, low-skill labor is involved. Surveys of the many federal minimum wage studies have concluded that the total demand for low-skill labor is relatively insensitive (inelastic), placing an estimate of (-.3) in the upper end of the likely range.[9] A major problem in using evidence from federal minimum wage studies, however, is that variation in the minimum wage relative to average wages has always been very small. In many industries, the labor cost increases implied by the mandate are larger than any that have been imposed by the federal minimum wage. Moreover, unlike the minimum wage, which if unindexed will decline relative to wages *over time* (if only through inflation), the impact of a mandate is driven by health care costs that may well increase relative to wages. Still another factor is that studies of the federal minimum wage have usually relied on aggregate time series data. It is extremely difficult to detect the effects of a change in the minimum wage on employment with such data, given the many other forces that are changing over time. Moreover, it is particularly difficult to estimate the long-run response to wage cost changes with time series data. Because a firm's options are limited in the short run—for example, replacing labor with capital takes time—the long-run response will be more elastic than the short run. Thus, there is a built-in downward bias in the federal minimum wage evidence. A number of recent studies of changes in state minimum wages have reported quite varied findings. Two highly publicized studies surveyed small samples of fast-food restaurants before and after the minimum was changed to estimate the employment impact of changes in a state minimum.[10] Both studies report no effect of the changed minimum on employment in the restaurants in their panels. Three other studies of state minimums use more traditional and more broadly representative data to implement their econometric models.[11] Two of these studies report negative impacts of changes in state minimums on employment; one study reports a response elasticity of (-.2), and the other reports a much more elastic response of (-1.0). The third study by David Card reports very small to no employment effect. The three studies based on large employment samples covering all low-wage industries and all employers appear much more reliable than the two studies based on small and select panels of employers.[12]

Other sources of evidence on response elasticities are the many econometric studies conducted over the years estimating the long-run elasticity of demand for labor. These studies frequently use variation in wage costs that arise cross-sectionally (for example, firms in the same industry but located in different parts of the country or in different countries and facing different labor costs) rather than using changes in minimum wage laws. Because cross-sectional differences in labor costs tend to be more permanent, differences in labor demand are more likely to reflect longer-term adjustments to the cost differentials. Summarizing the results of these empirical studies, Ronald Ehrenberg and Robert Smith conclude that changes in labor costs economywide appear to be associated with a total response elasticity that could be as high as (-.75). Among particular industries, the various studies reviewed show estimates that range from (-.3) in U.S. manufacturing to a range of (-.34) to (-1.20) across individual industries in retailing.[13] In a summary of over 100 studies of the elasticity of demand in individual industries, Daniel Hamermesh finds a "medium range" value of about (-1.0) considering both substitution and scale effects.[14]

Studies of the size of consumer responses to changes in prices of products and services are also relevant for judging the size of the employment response to a mandate in the industries we have identified as strongly affected. In these industries, costs and, therefore, prices would be sharply increased. Studies show that the consumer product "purchased meals" has a high price elasticity of demand (-2.3), meaning that for each percentage point increase in the price, consumers will reduce their purchases of meals away from home by 2.3 percent.[15] This is important evidence that the "eating and drinking" industry, one of the most highly affected, will have a large total response elasticity. The private household services industry is also likely to have a high consumer response elasticity. Like the restaurant industry, it provides a service for which fairly good substitutes are readily available, that is, "do it yourself."

Our review of the literature suggests that the range (-.2) to (-.5) likely contains the true value of the response elasticity for the economy as a whole. In this study, we use an estimate of (-.3) to generate the economy-wide effects of the mandate on job displacement, although significant differences in elasticities may be expected in certain heavily affected industries, such as retailing and personal services.[16]

Effects on Employment

Some 130 million persons worked during 1992, and of this group approximately 111 million wage-and-salary workers would have been subject to the Clinton employer mandate had it been in effect. The total effect of the plan would differ greatly according to a worker's premandate insurance status. The cost of employing a worker who is uninsured would unambiguously rise under the mandate, while wage costs for employers who already cover their workers would likely decline on average, although as described below there would be individual losses as well as gains within the covered sector. We have conducted separate analyses for the 45 million uninsured workers (many of whom are covered through other means as shown in table 1) and for the 66 million already insured by their employers.

The characteristics of workers differ considerably by insurance status (table 3). Uninsured workers are about seven times more likely to be part time, and they work close to five weeks less than insured workers during the year. They are much more likely to be high school dropouts and much less likely to be college graduates. About 20 percent of the uninsured are younger than age twenty-five compared with 7 percent of the insured. A much larger proportion of the insured are married men than the uninsured (39 percent versus 23 percent), while married women and single men make up a larger share of the uninsured. (Close to two-thirds of married women without employer coverage are covered by their husband's employer policy.) On average, the annual earnings of workers who are not insured by their employers are less than half the earnings of workers with employer-provided insurance.

In sum, workers who currently do not receive insurance from their employers have characteristics associated with relatively low skills and worker productivity, and they have relatively low wages. A mandate requiring employers to purchase an insurance policy for these workers would significantly increase the cost of employing them. If the Clinton mandate had been implemented without any employer subsidies in 1993, the average annual premium cost per worker for employees in the uninsured sector would have been $1,923 (assuming Hewitt Associates' estimates of premium prices and prorating costs for part-time, part-year workers). A premium of this size would have added 13 percent to the average annual wage (table 4).

Wage cost increases would have been considerably higher in certain

TABLE 3
CHARACTERISTICS OF WAGE-AND-SALARY WORKERS
COVERED BY THE MANDATE, BY INSURANCE STATUS WITH
CURRENT EMPLOYER

Type of Worker	Uninsured	Insured
Number of workers (million)	45.1	66.1
Percent part-time (<30 hours)	22.9	3.4
Average weeks worked in the year	44.8	49.5
Percent high school dropout	20.5	8.0
Percent college graduate	16.6	30.8
Percent less than age 25	19.9	6.9
Annual earnings (1993 dollars)	14,962	31,220
Family type (percent)		
Two-parent family	32.3	33.3
Couple, no child	24.3	28.9
Single parent	5.5	6.2
Individual	37.9	31.6
Gender and marital status (percent)		
Woman, married	33.3	22.5
Woman, not married	19.8	20.0
Man, married	23.2	39.4
Man, not married	23.6	17.9

NOTE: Workers' demographic characteristics are measured at the time of the survey in March 1993. Insurance status refers to coverage during calendar year 1992; earnings and work experience also refer to 1992. Earnings were adjusted for estimated wage growth between 1992 and 1993.
SOURCES: March 1993 CPS.

industries. Without employer subsidies, the mandate would boost wage costs for full-time workers by 22 percent in the eating and drinking industry, 16 percent in "other retail," 20 percent in agriculture, and 19 percent in personal services. The provision of employer subsidies would reduce the cost increase generated by the mandate, although wage costs for uninsured workers would still rise by 8.5 percent on the whole. It is the exclusion from the premium subsidy of the entire public sector (until the year 2001) and of firms with 5,000 or more workers until the year 2000 that accounts for the continuing cost pressure of the mandate, even when the premium caps are implemented in the subsidized sectors.

Effects among Currently Uninsured Workers. In assessing the effect of the Clinton mandate on jobs for currently uninsured workers, we employ

TABLE 4
PREDICTED CHANGE IN EMPLOYER PREMIUM ATTRIBUTABLE
TO IMPLEMENTATION OF CLINTON MANDATE,
BY PREMANDATE INSURANCE STATUS
(dollars)

	Uninsured	Insured	All Workers
Employer's average annual premium cost per worker			
Before mandate	0	2,660	1,580
After implementation, without premium cap	1,936	2,495	2,268
After implementation, with premium cap	1,268	2,403	1,942
Change from before mandate to after implementation with cap	1,268	−258	362
Average annual wage and salary income of workers before mandate	14,962	31,220	24,616

NOTE: Based on 1993 premium costs, wages, and insurance status.
SOURCE: Estimates use Hewitt Associates premium costs (see table 2). Employer share of premium is estimated based on Clinton plan assignment of full-time and part-time status and rules for prorating premiums for part-time work. The premiums of part-year workers are prorated for actual weeks worked, which is the period of employer liability. Simulations use the March 1993 CPS.

alternative assumptions of premium prices, the extent of wage shifting and wage elasticity. We also present two sets of estimates. In one, we assume no subsidy for employers to reduce the cost effect of the mandate. In the other, we use the subsidy structure detailed in the Clinton plan.

Table 5 shows the job loss that could be expected without subsidies. Estimates are presented assessing both moderate shifting (70 percent of cost increases are passed to wages) and "maximum" shifting (an 80 percent cost shift). Under the 80 percent shift assumption, where premium cost increases are shifted down to the legal minimum, the aggregate job loss would range from 300,000 to 2.3 million, depending on the assumptions concerning response elasticities and premium prices (table 5). When the less extreme wage-shifting assumption is assumed, the job loss esti-

TABLE 5

ESTIMATED JOB LOSS AMONG UNINSURED WORKERS UNDER AN EMPLOYER MANDATE WITHOUT EMPLOYER SUBSIDIES, UNDER DIFFERENT ASSUMPTIONS OF PREMIUM COSTS, WAGE SHIFTING, AND EMPLOYER RESPONSE (ELASTICITY)

(thousands of workers)

Source of Premium Cost[a]	Moderate shifting[b] 100% shifting of premium cost to workers down to $6.50/hour[b]			Maximum shifting 100% shifting of premium cost to workers down to $4.50/hour[b]		
Elasticity	0.1	0.3	0.5	0.1	0.3	0.5
Administration	509	1,527	2,545	324	973	1,621
Foster-Higgins Survey	727	2,182	3,636	463	1,390	2,316

a. See table 2 for the premium prices associated with the sources specified.

b. For workers earning at or below $6.50 (4.25) per hour there is no shifting and cost rises by the full cost of the insurance. Partial shifting begins after $6.50 (4.25) and equals the amount by which the worker's weekly earnings exceed $6.50 (4.25) times his weekly hours. The cost of these workers to their employers rises by only a fraction of their insurance cost. Full shifting is reached when weekly earnings exceed the weekly premium amount plus $6.50 (4.25) times weekly hours. The cost of employing these workers does not rise at all as a consequence of the mandate.

SOURCE: Estimates based on a microsimulation using the March 1993 Current Population Survey (CPS). Wages and premiums were adjusted to 1993 levels and premium costs were assigned to workers based on their family type and hours and weeks worked. Simulations were applied to the population of wage and salary workers covered by the Clinton mandate.

13

TABLE 6
COMPARISON OF THE NUMBER OF UNINSURED WORKERS DISPLACED UNDER THE CLINTON MANDATE WITH EMPLOYER SUBSIDIES, USING DIFFERENT ASSUMPTIONS OF PREMIUM COSTS, CAP LEVELS, AND COST SHIFTING
(thousands)

Moderate Cost Shift

| Premium Source | Total All Sectors[a] | | Subsidized Sector[a] | | Unsubsidized Sector | |
| | | | | | Firms with < 5,000 workers | Public Sector |
	Cap I[b]	Cap II[c]	Cap I[b]	Cap II[c]		
Administration	642.7	749.6	295.8	402.7	280.2	66.7
Hewitt Associates	780.7	887.6	295.8	402.7	384.7	100.2
Foster Higgins	782.4	889.3	295.8	402.7	388.4	98.2

Moderate Cost Shift

Premium Source	Total All Sectors[a]		Subsidized Sector[a]		Unsubsidized Sector	
	Cap I[b]	Cap II[c]	Cap I[b]	Cap II[c]	Firms with < 5,000 workers	Public Sector
Administration	418.3	493.9	210.8	286.4	164.6	42.9
Hewitt Associates	519.6	595.2	210.8	286.4	245.9	62.9
Foster Higgins	525.1	600.7	210.8	286.4	250.4	63.9

NOTE: In the subsidized sector, the cost of insurance is the firm's premium cost cap (expressed as a fraction) times the worker's wage, unless the firm's cap amount (cap fraction times annual wage bill) is greater than its total annual premium cost. In this case the insurance cost equals the actual premium cost. Moderate cost shifting in the subsidized sector means shifting 100 percent of the insurance cost to workers with wages above $300 per week, shifting one-half the cost to workers with wages below $300 a week, but no shifting to workers earning below $6.50 an hour. Maximum cost shifting in the subsidized sector follows the same pattern, but does not stop shifting until workers earning minimumwage are reached—$4.25 per hour. See table 5 for the shifting methodology used in the uninsured sectors. For basic annual premium without caps, see table 2.

a. Cap assumption I is based on the schedule of premium caps by firm size and average annual wage threshold given in the Health Security Act, Section 6123 (see table 9). Assumption II illustrates the case where inflation erodes the wage threshold levels so that all firms face the 7.9% maximum.

b. Based on 1993 wages and firm size.

c. All firms at 7.9 cap.

TABLE 7
PAYROLL CAP PERCENTAGES FOR LIMITING OUTLAYS
ON PREMIUM COSTS
(percent)

Average Wage[a]	Less than 25 Employees[b]	25-50 Employees	50-75 Employee
Less than $12,000	3.5	4.4	5.3
$12-15,000	4.4	5.3	6.2
$15-18,000	5.3	6.2	7.1
$18-21,000	6.2	7.1	7.9
$21-24,000	7.1	7.9	7.9
More than $24,000	7.9	7.9	7.9

a. Average annual full-time equivalent wage.
b. Average number of full-time equivalent employees.
SOURCE: Health Security Act, Section 6123.

mates increase significantly, ranging from a low of 500,000 up to 3.6 million depending on the premium cost and elasticity assumptions chosen. Under what we believe to be reasonable assumptions—the Foster Higgins premium costs, an elasticity of (-.3) and moderate (70 percent) cost shifting—the job loss without premium subsidies would be 2.2 million among the uninsured workers covered by the mandate.

Table 6 displays estimates of the disemployment generated by the Clinton employer mandate, assuming that the subsidy scheme specified in Section 6123 of the Health Security Act is implemented. It is important to keep in mind that under the current plan, significant numbers of low-wage uninsured workers are not subsidized, at least not for the foreseeable future. Firms with more than 5,000 employees are excluded from the employer subsidy program until the fifth year of the plan, at which time subsidies for this group would begin to be phased in, while the entire public sector would first become eligible for subsidies in the year 2002.

In the subsidized sector, the employer's premium costs are limited to a specified percentage of wages, and the percentage varies with the average wage (per full-time equivalent employee) and the size of the firm, ranging from a low of 3.5 percent to a maximum of 7.9 percent (table 7). Table 6 includes estimates of a situation in which all firms in the subsidized sector are at the maximum premium cap of 7.9 percent (see Cap Assumption II). This is not an idle curiosity, since no provision is made for indexing the wage thresholds; as a result, firms will move closer and closer to the maximum cap of 7.9 percent each year as inflation raises workers' wages. Cap Assumption I refers to the full array of cap percentages indicated in the Clinton plan.

We estimate that if Cap Assumption I were implemented, the number of jobs lost because of the mandate would fall to approximately 780,000, assuming Foster Higgins premium prices and moderate cost shifting. (The Hewitt premium prices produce almost identical results.) If we assume the maximum possible cost shifting (down to the minimum wage), these estimates are reduced to about 520,000. When we substitute the administration's estimate of premium prices, displacement effects are lower: 643,000 jobs lost with moderate shifting and 418,000 with maximum shifting. If inflation raises the premium cap to 7.9 percent in all subsidized firms (Cap Assumption II), the job loss would increase to 890,000, assuming that the higher premium prices of Hewitt or Foster Higgins are the correct ones and that moderate cost shifting prevails. In all cases, however, it is the unsubsidized sector that contributes the major portion of the job loss.

It is clear that without subsidies the Clinton mandate has the potential for creating a serious disruption in the labor market for low-skill workers. The disruption would be especially severe in certain industries, as shown in table 8. This potential is important to keep in mind because of the uncertainty that is likely to surround the implementation of any employer subsidy program. The employer subsidies are a "capped" entitlement, since they are subject to a federal expenditure limitation requiring congressional action to be lifted. If firms in heavily affected industries doubt that full appropriations will be forthcoming, they may react as if there were no subsidies, and the estimates of job displacement without subsidies would become highly relevant.

But even assuming that the employer subsidy program functions as planned, the mandate will generate job losses and in amounts that cannot be regarded as trivial. As shown in table 8, the job loss will be concentrated in particular industries. The extent of disemployment is likely to be greater in the near term than the numbers we have generated would suggest, because wages probably cannot be reduced immediately to absorb the increase in employer costs, at least not to the extent we have assumed.

Effects in the Covered Sector. Firms that currently insure their workers, on balance, are likely to experience reductions in premium costs under the Clinton mandate because: (1) the premium subsidies would reduce costs to firms with high ratios of premium costs to wages; (2) the employer's contribution would decline for workers who had formerly opted for family coverage since the plan calls for the employer share of family premiums to be divided among employers of husbands and wives (see table 2). The extent of the premium decline is greater for married workers without children and for single parents who are charged at a lower rate under the plan than married workers with children. Employers of married workers or single parents, however, who under the current system carry only individual coverage, will experience *cost increases* since all workers must be assigned

TABLE 8
Estimates of Job Loss by Industry under the Clinton Mandate, Comparing Effects with and without Premium Caps and by Assumption about Size of Premium
(thousands of workers)

Industry	Without Premium Caps		With Premium Caps	
	Administration premium costs	Hewitt Assoc. premium costs	Administration premium costs	Hewitt Assoc. premium costs
Eating and drinking	402.3	545.0	169.7	207.3
Other retailing	374.7	517.0	182.6	229.6
Construction	66.9	95.9	24.0	24.6
Agriculture	83.7	117.0	18.3	19.2
Business services	42.1	60.3	16.8	18.4
Personal services	105.8	147.0	34.4	39.7
Educational services	50.2	75.7	40.5	60.2
Transportation, communications, and public utilities	21.7	32.4	11.4	14.3
Health services (excluding hospitals)	38.2	56.9	17.4	18.9
Wholesale trade	18.8	27.9	7.6	8.3
Repair services	28.1	39.0	9.3	9.8
Insurance and real estate	14.1	21.0	5.8	6.5
Household workers	91.1	124.0	10.9	10.9
Other professional	11.0	15.6	4.6	4.3
Public administration	12.5	18.2	12.5	18.2
Hospital	8.4	12.4	6.2	7.7
Rest of economy	157.5	231.4	71.5	82.6
Total	1,527.1	2,136.7	642.7	780.7

NOTE: For methodology and data used see notes to tables 5 and 6.

the family rate that corresponds to their family status under the Clinton plan and the family rate always exceeds the individual rate.[17] Taking account of these basic factors, we estimate that premium costs among insured workers would have declined by $258 on average for the year had the plan been in effect in 1993. Since the compensation of insured workers averaged $33,880 in 1993 ($31,220 in cash wages and $2,660 in health benefits), the premium reduction would reduce total compensation costs by 0.76 percent. We anticipate that most of the reduction in premium costs would be passed on to workers in the form of increases in money wages. No obstacle such as the minimum wage impedes wage increases. Moreover, among these relatively high-wage workers, we would expect a highly inelastic supply of labor. Assuming a supply elasticity of (.03) and a demand elasticity of (-.3), the Clinton plan would result in an employment increase of about 15,000 in the covered sector, which is hardly any offset to the 780,000 job loss expected in the uncovered sector.

Distributional Effects

The effect of the Clinton plan on workers' incomes would take two forms. One is the wage loss (or gain) that would result from the shifting of increases (or decreases) in premiums generated by the implementation of the plan. The other is the loss in income accompanying the job loss that is also generated by the mandate. Those who lose their jobs would likely experience the greatest reductions in income, but it is difficult to identify who precisely they would be or to quantify the income loss involved.

The effect on workers' earnings from the shifting of premium cost changes under the mandate can be simulated, and the results of such a simulation are displayed in table 9. Two sets of estimates are given. One employs the "moderate shift" assumption (premiums are shifted to wages down to $6.50 per hour); the other employs the "maximum shift" assumption (all premium cost increases are shifted down to the minimum wage of $4.25). Both estimates use premium costs that reflect the employer subsidies.

Premium cost changes are predictably much larger and always negative for uninsured workers. Under the moderate shift assumption, uninsured workers would see their annual wages of $14,962 decline by $873 after implementation of the mandate, a 5.8 percent wage loss. Under the maximum degree of shifting that might occur in the long run, the wages of these workers would fall by $990, a 6.6 percent loss.

Some workers currently insured by their employers would also experience wage reductions, but a majority would experience wage gains. On average, we estimate a gain of $272 annually for those who are already insured by their employers, less than a 1 percent increase from their relatively high premandate wage of $31,220. Combining all workers—the currently insured and the uninsured—wages on balance fall by about 1 percent.

The total changes in income conceal larger shifts within both the

TABLE 9
AVERAGE ANNUAL EARNINGS OF WAGE-AND-SALARY WORKERS IN 1993 AND SIMULATED EARNINGS AFTER IMPLEMENTATION OF THE CLINTON MANDATE WITH PREMIUM CAPS, BY WAGE SHIFTING ASSUMPTION
(dollars)

	Moderate Shifting of Premium				Maximum Shifting of Premium			
	Earnings before mandate	Earnings post mandate	Change		Earnings before mandate	Earnings post mandate	Change	
			Dollars	Percent			Dollars	Percent
All eligible workers	24,616	24,422	-194	-0.8	24,616	24,372	-244	-1.0
Not currently insured by employer	14,962	14,089	-873	-5.8	14,962	13,972	-990	-6.6
Currently insured by employer	31,220	31,492	272	0.9	31,220	31,487	267	0.9

NOTE: Under moderate shifting premium cost increases are shifted to workers through wage reductions at wages of $300 a week or more with partial shift below $300 and no shifting below $6.50 per hour. With maximum shifting premium costs are shifted to wages down to the minimum wage.

SOURCE: The estimates are derived from microsimulations using the March 1993 Current Population Survey with wages adjusted to 1993 levels. The wage reductions are estimated as shifted components of the employer's share of the annual 1993 premium based on Hewitt premium prices. Each worker's annual premium varies with his/her family status, weeks and hours worked as well as on the estimated average earnings and the size of the worker's firm (which determines the premium subsidies).

TABLE 10
EFFECTS OF THE CLINTON MANDATE ON ANNUAL WAGES
AND THE RISK OF JOB LOSS, BY PREMANDATE INSURANCE STATUS

| | Uninsured | | | Insured | |
	At risk of job loss; no wage reduction	Wages reduced; little or no job loss	Wages reduced	Wages increased	No wage change
Number of workers (000's)	19,923	25,205	12,825	40,269	12,887
Likely job loss (000's)	781	a	a	a	a
Annual wages premandate ($)	6,172	21,900	39,516	29,807	28,957
Annual wages postmandate ($)	6,172	20,347	38,368	30,601	28,957
Change in wage					
Dollars	a	(1,563)	(1,148)	794	0
Percent	a	-7.1	-2.9	2.7	0

NOTE: These estimates assume moderate shifting (down to $6.50 per hour) and use capped premiums (based on Hewitt premium prices) with employer subsidies as specified in the plan.
a. Employment change is negligible.
SOURCE: The estimates are derived from microsimulations using the March 1993 Current Population Survey with wages adjusted to 1993 levels. The wage reductions are estimated as shifted components of the employer's share of the annual 1993 premium based on Hewitt premium prices. Each worker's annual premium varies with his or her family status, weeks and hours worked as well as on the estimated average earnings and the size of the worker's firm (which determine the premium subsidies).

uninsured and the insured sectors. Within the uninsured sector, the job loss generated by the mandate involves mainly the lowest-wage workers, whose wages cannot readily be rolled back to compensate for the new premium costs. As shown in table 10, close to 20 million workers with average annual earnings of $6,172 would become vulnerable to job loss, assuming that employers could not easily reduce the wages of those earning less than $6.50 per hour. We have estimated that 780,000 of these low-wage workers (3.9 percent) would likely lose their jobs. Uninsured workers who earn above the $6.50 per hour level diminish their risk of job loss through wage reductions. Their average annual wage of $21,900 before

TABLE 11
ESTIMATED SHIFTING EFFECT OF THE CLINTON MANDATE ON THE ANNUAL
EARNINGS OF UNINSURED WORKERS, BY TYPE
(1993 wages and premium prices)

Workers	Number of workers (millions)	Earnings in premandate dollars (mean)	Earnings Reduction	
			Dollars	As % of premandate earnings
All workers	25.2	21,910	1,563	7.1
Women	12.5	18,364	1,383	7.5
Men	12.7	25,384	1,739	6.9
Married parent	9.4	23,695	1,910	8.1
Married, no child	7.3	24,745	1,666	6.7
Single parent	1.0	17,728	1,222	6.9
Individual	7.4	17,425	1,067	6.1
Annual earnings				
<$12,500	7.6	7,202	463	6.4
$12,500–25,000	9.8	18,208	1,423	7.8
$25,000	7.8	41,402	2,822	6.8

NOTE: Under the moderate wage shifting assumption, the premium is shifted to the worker through wage reductions down to $6.50 an hour.
SOURCE: The estimates are derived from microsimulations using the March 1993 Current Population Survey with wages adjusted to 1993 levels. The wage reductions are estimated as shifted components of the employer's share of the annual 1993 premium based on Hewitt premium prices. Each worker's annual premium varies with his or her family status, weeks and hours worked as well as on the estimated average earnings and the size of the worker's firm, which determine the premium subsidies.

the mandate would fall by $1,563 on average, a decline of 7.1 percent.

Among workers already insured by their employers, about 40 million would experience wage gains averaging $794 per year, because the premium their employers pay would decline. Another 12.8 million would find their wages reduced by an average amount of $1,148 per year because of premium increases,[18] while an additional 12.9 million would not experience a change in either premiums or wages. Insured workers experiencing wage reductions have higher earnings than those with wage gains or no change. But insured workers in any category are a higher-income group than the uninsured who experience either job loss or relatively large wage losses.

Among the uninsured who would retain their jobs at the expense of

TABLE 12

ESTIMATED FEDERAL EMPLOYER SUBSIDIES UNDER THE CLINTON MANDATE
IF IMPLEMENTED IN 1993 BEFORE AND AFTER WAGE SHIFTING,
ALTERNATIVE ESTIMATES BASED ON DIFFERENT PREMIUM PRICES
(millions of dollars)

	Administration	Hewitt Assoc.	Foster Higgins
Before wage shifting	14,058	38,318	37,530
After wage shifting	15,925	40,107	39,319

NOTE: Because of data limitations we lack direct observations on the average wage per full-time equivalent worker in the individual worker's firm. The relevant firm level wage was estimated for aggregations of firms by firm size and industry, and all firms in each size and industry category were assumed to have the same average wage.

SOURCE: The estimates are based on the March 1993 Current Population Survey (CPS) with wages and premium prices adjusted to 1993 levels. The number of workers as reported in the CPS's 1000+ category that are in firms with less than 5,000 workers (who are elegible for the subsidy) was estimated by extrapolating the detailed size class by industry data given in the Census Bureau's *Enterprise Statistics*.

wage reductions, no clear pattern of losses emerges either by wage level, by gender, or by family or marital status (table 11). Women would experience somewhat greater relative losses than men, and married parents (particularly married women) would experience somewhat greater reductions than other groups.

The Clinton mandate is not likely to produce progressive redistributive effects among the working population. In fact, the concentration of job losses and wage reductions at the bottom of the earnings distribution suggests quite the opposite. Because the employer subsidies are based on the average wage in the firm rather than the individual worker's wage, these large federal expenditures are not well targeted and frequently lead to capricious outcomes

What Will Federal Subsidies to Employers and Workers Cost?

The Clinton plan reduces the negative impact of the mandate on employment and earnings by providing a system of employer subsidies funded by the federal government. Subsidies are also to be paid to low-income workers to help defray the family share of the premium and the family's liability during periods of nonwork. Finally, low-income families with no covered workers are to receive subsidies to help them pay the premiums charged by the health alliances. Our estimates of the federal budget expenditures needed to fund these subsidies are based on what the costs

TABLE 13
ESTIMATED EMPLOYER SUBSIDIES BY INDUSTRY AND PREMIUM ASSUMPTION
AFTER WAGE SHIFTING
(in millions of dollars)

Industry	Clinton Plan Premiums	Foster Higgins Premiums	Hewitt Associates Premiums
Eating and drinking	2,728	4,727	4,663
Other retail	2,933	6,658	6,753
Construction	643	2,332	2,463
Agriculture	1,044	1,924	1,970
Business services	715	1,735	1,742
Personal services	1,216	2,275	2,253
Educational services	269	763	798
Transportation, communications, and public utilities	396	1,379	1,438
Health services (excluding hospitals)	956	3,038	3,032
Wholesale trade	328	1,143	1,206
Repair services	429	1,036	1,064
Insurance and real estate	276	840	882
Household workers	762	1,128	1,109
Other professional	0	237	261
Hospital	64	881	899
Rest of economy	3,168	9,222	9,575
Total	15,925	39,319	40,107

SOURCE: See table 12.

would have been if the plan had been in effect in 1993. We estimate a total cost for these subsidies of $79.5 billion.

Employer Subsidies. The employer subsidy varies from firm to firm and is based on the difference between an employer's total premium costs and a capped amount that is not to exceed a certain percentage of the firm's payroll. The capped percentages are displayed in table 7, and as shown they increase with firm size and with the firm's average annual wage per full-time equivalent worker. The maximum that a firm would be required to pay for premiums is set at 7.9 percent of wages, except for firms with more than 5,000 workers and all government employees. The large firms in the alliances first become eligible in the fifth year of the plan, when they would get a partial subsidy (rising to a full subsidy by the eighth year); the public sector begins to receive subsidies in the year 2002.

As shown in table 12, our estimates suggest that the Clinton health plan, had it been in effect in 1993, would have required a federal outlay of about $40 billion, after taking account of wage shifting. This figure is based on the premium prices estimated by Hewitt Associates. Our estimates do not change significantly when we substitute the premium levels obtained from Foster Higgins data, but they change dramatically when the administration's assumptions about premium costs are employed, falling to only $16 billion. Obviously, estimates of the budget consequences of the Clinton mandate are highly sensitive to the estimator's assumption of what the premium price will be for the basic insurance package.

More than 80 percent of the federal subsidy to employers would be paid to firms that currently do not insure their workers; but this still leaves a sizable subsidy ($6.6 billion) that must be paid to firms that are now providing insurance. The subsidies would be concentrated in industries with smaller firms and lower wage rates. Eating and drinking and other retail industries would receive 28 percent of all subsidies (table 13).

By how much would employer subsidies grow over time if the plan were implemented? As explained above, because the wage thresholds are not indexed for inflation, the premium caps will move to the ceiling of 7.9 percent in all firms as inflation raises the money wages paid. This would reduce the federal employer subsidy by about 15 percent; but as we showed above, it would also lead to increased job loss. Other factors would operate in the direction of increasing the subsidy. Premium prices may well continue to increase faster than wages even if the rate of increase were to slow, reflecting the historical pattern for health care expenditures to rise faster than income in the United States, as in most other countries. This would be a factor generating increases in the federal employer subsidy, unless stringent national price controls were adopted. It is debatable, however, whether such controls could be maintained over the long term, given the demand of the public for more and better-quality health care.

Higher premiums may also be generated by changes in the distribution of workers across firms and industries in response to the subsidies themselves. As discussed below, firms would have a strong incentive to organize production so that low-wage workers are together with other low-wage workers and high-wage workers with other high-wage workers.

Subsidies to Low-Income Workers. Workers and their families are directly responsible for paying to the alliances 20 percent of the annual premium cost—the "family share"—and they are liable for the full premium cost (employer and family share) during periods of the year that they are out of the labor force or unemployed, when no employer contribution would be made. Part-time workers also owe the difference between the prorated employer premium and the full employer share. Federal subsidies are provided to families according to a sliding scale

25

TABLE 14
FEDERAL SUBSIDIES TO LOW-INCOME WORKERS AND NONWORKERS
AND THEIR FAMILIES IN THE CLINTON HEALTH PLAN
(dollars, in millions)

Work Category	Number of Families with Subsidy (millions)		Subsidies for Family Share (dollars)	Subsidies for Unfunded Liabilities (dollars)	Total Combined Subsidy (dollars)
	Family share	Unfunded liability			
Low-income workers	18.6	11.9	6,561	8,715	15,276
Low-income nonworkers	10.2	10.8	4,451	19,743	24,194
Total workers and nonworkers	28.8	22.7	11,012	18,458	39,470

NOTE: Excludes any who were receiving Medicare or Medicaid.
SOURCE: Based on microsimulation using the March 1993 Current Population Survey. Subsidies were calculated based on the provisions in the Clinton plan which phase out subsidies as income increases and they are based on Hewitt premium prices.

based on income. Those whose incomes fall below $1,000 receive full subsidies, and the subsidy starts to decline when income exceeds $1,000. It falls to zero when income reaches 150 percent of the poverty line in the case of the family share and to 250 percent of the poverty line in the case of the unfunded liability.

The total cost of the subsidies to working families would have been $20 billion if the plan had been in effect in 1993, but $4.7 billion of these subsidies would be paid to Medicaid and Medicare recipients. While federal expenditures on Medicaid and Medicare would decline as a result of these groups' participation in the health plan, it is extremely difficult to determine the extent of the decline. We handle the problem by subtracting out the subsidies to Medicare and Medicaid recipients, leaving a net subsidy to low-income families of $15 billion (table 14).

Subsidies to Nonworkers. Nonworkers and their families are eligible for subsidies to help them pay for both the 20 percent of the premium that is specified as the worker's share and the 80 percent that employers directly forward to the alliances. Subsidies are also provided to help with the copayments that are part of the insurance plans obtained, but we do not estimate their cost.

Nonworkers include some early retirees, but they are mostly individuals who, for a variety of reasons, have not worked for an extended period of time. About 11.5 million persons who did not work at all in 1992 reported themselves to the Current Population Survey as "unrelated individuals," which means they were not living with another family member. This group reported very low incomes and probably did not contain many early retirees. There were also 1.4 million couples who reported no work in 1992 and have considerably higher incomes; this group probably did contain some early retirees.

The Clinton plan's subsidy scheme treats early retirees differently (more generously) from other nonworkers. Our data do not allow us to identify early retirees, so we treated all our nonworkers as if they were not early retirees. This means that our estimates will be slightly downward based.

Table 14 shows that $24.1 billion in subsidies would have been required for all nonworkers, if the Clinton plan had been in effect in 1993. The bulk of this subsidy goes to the unrelated individual group.

Effects on Resource Allocation

While the employer subsidy in the Clinton plan would reduce the job loss created by the mandate, it would also open the door to a reallocation of labor resources that could significantly reduce the productivity of our economy. The inefficiencies created are potentially of greater importance than the job losses associated with mandates or the more obvious budget costs required to finance the subsidies.[19]

Problems arise under the subsidy scheme for several reasons, but the fundamental one is that the cost of insurance for any single worker depends on the level of his or her wage *and* the wage level of all the coworkers in his or her firm. Two features of the subsidy scheme contribute to this result. One is that in small firms—firms with less than seventy-five workers—the payroll cap and therefore the cost of insurance fall with the average wage of the firm and the size of the firm below the seventy-five-worker level (see table 9). Thus the annual cost of insuring a worker earning $15,000 per year in a firm with sixty employees and an average wage of $24,000 would be $1,185, since such a firm would have a cap of 7.9 percent;[20] yet the cost of insuring the same worker in the same size firm but one with an average wage of $10,000 would be $795 since such a firm has a cap of 5.3 percent. And the cost of the same $15,000-a-year worker would fall to $525 if this firm reduced its employment below twenty-five employees, since the cap then falls to 3.5 percent. A powerful incentive is surely created for low-wage industries to reduce their firm size and for higher-wage firms to contract out the functions of low-skill workers to small specialized firms.

The perverse incentive to separate skilled and unskilled workers does not depend solely on the variable cap feature of the subsidy scheme for smaller firms. Even if all firms faced a cap of 7.9 percent, it will generally be the case that a firm employing both highly skilled and unskilled workers would be able to reduce its total insurance costs by separating its workers into two firms, one with high-wage workers and the other with low-wage workers. The savings arise because high-skill workers are likely to cost less to insure when the firm pays the actual premium cost rather than the capped percentage of wages: 7.9 percent of an annual wage of $50,000 ($3,950) typically exceeds the actual premium cost. But low-skill workers will generally be less expensive to insure when the percentage cap is applied: 7.9 percent of $10,000 ($790) will almost certainly be less than the actual premium cost.

The savings from separating workers can be considerable. Suppose, for example, that a firm with 200 workers employs 100 skilled workers each earning $40,000 a year and 100 unskilled workers earning $10,000, so the average wage would be $25,000. If the actual premium cost per worker is $2,000, the firm would pay the capped amount of $1,975 (.079 x $25,000) because on average it is lower. The total insurance costs for the 200 workers combined in one firm would then be $395,500 ($1,975 x 200). But with a cap of 7.9 percent, insurance for each high-wage worker is costing the firm $3,160 (.079 x $40,000), $1,160 more per worker than the $2,000 per worker actual premium cost. By separating the 100 high-wage workers into their own firm, the business would save $116,000 on these workers' insurance costs ($1,160 x 100). The low-wage workers would continue to cost 7.9 percent of their $10,000 wage, $790 per worker, or $79,000 for the 100 workers. As a consequence of segregation, total costs of insuring these 200 workers would fall from $395,000 to $279,000—a 30 percent saving.

It is difficult to predict the extent to which firms would engage in this kind of subsidy gamesmanship or to imagine all the strategies that might be pursued. As long as the insurance savings from segregating workers by skill outweigh the costs of segregation, firms will segregate. And as long as the insurance cost reductions from forming smaller firms with lower caps exceeds the cost disadvantage of smaller size, smaller firms will be formed at the expense of large ones.

Companies with 5,000 or more workers that are not eligible for any premium cap for the first four years would have a particularly strong incentive to form smaller units, especially if they employ low-wage workers. As Alan Krueger notes, firms such as McDonald's, which have both company-owned and franchised stores, would have an incentive to promote franchises that would be treated as small businesses eligible for the small business premium cap and shift out of company-owned stores.[21] The firm size of McDonald's (and many other retail chains) exceeds the 5,000 level, so the company-owned stores would have no cap.

Through the contracting out of services or goods that employ low-skill workers, the insurance cost advantages of small size and segregation by wage level could be obtained. One would anticipate that services such as cleaning and clerical work or the manufacture of particular kinds of parts would increasingly become contracted work.

The reorganization of activities prompted solely by the pressure to reduce insurance costs is bound to reduce efficiency, leading to a misallocation of resources and reduced productivity. In addition, one can anticipate negative consequences for workers stemming from an increase in segregation. Internal mobility within the firm is typically attained through on-the-job training, which is partially funded by the workers themselves by taking lower wages. The increased insurance cost of combining low-wage and high-wage workers will therefore discourage training. Moreover, the mandate itself will discourage training in very large firms that are not eligible for any subsidy since insurance costs in these firms would greatly add to training costs.

Concluding Comments

Free health benefits like free lunches are wishful thinking. There is no way to extend health insurance coverage to millions of people without paying for it. The employer mandate put forth in the Clinton health plan appears to us to be a poor way to pay the health bill. True, it would guarantee insurance to 18 million workers who now lack it. But this insurance will not be a gift, as the workers themselves will be compelled to pay for it through lower wages, and were wage rollbacks are infeasible, through reductions in employment.

The employer subsidies added to the Clinton mandate would reduce the share of the bill paid through the employer, and therefore they would ameliorate job loss and wage rollbacks. But the subsidies are not large enough to eliminate job loss and wage rollbacks, which remain significant. The subsidies also come at a price. In addition to increasing budget expenditures by $40 billion, the subsidy scheme generates inefficient reorganization of business, creating peculiar incentives to form small firms and to segregate high-skill and low-skill workers. These market distortions would not be present if increased health coverage were provided to low-income families through direct subsidies rather than through an employer mandate.

Notes

1. Workers are exempt from the mandate if they work less than ten hours a week or if they are under the age of eighteen or are full-time, unmarried students under the age of twenty-four.

2. This phrase was used by Hillary Rodham Clinton in a speech to the American Hospital Association in August 1993, and it has been echoed frequently by other administration officials and representatives.

3. See testimony of Hewitt Associates by Dale H. Yamamoto, F.S.A., and Frank B. McArdle, *Pricing of the Standard Benefit Package in the Health Security Act*, U.S. House Subcommittee on Health and the Environment, Committee on Energy and Commerce, November 22, 1993.

4. Lewin-VHI estimates that the community-rated premium required by the plan would increase per person health costs for workers and their dependents by 14 percent (Lewin-VHI, Inc., *The Financial Impact of the Health Security Act*, December 9, 1993).

5. Existing studies of the size of the cost-shift factor are not conclusive. A study by the Congressional Budget Office (CBO) found a significant shift factor, while two other studies found no evidence for significant cost shifting. See *Responses to Uncompensated Care and Public Program Controls on Spending: Do Hospitals "Cost Shift"?* Congressional Budget Office, May, 1993; Michael A. Morrissey, *Cost Shifting in Health Care: Separating Evidence from Rhetoric* (Paper prepared for the American Enterprise Institute, Washington, D.C., Sept. 18, 1993); and Jack Hadley and Judith Feder, "Hospital Cost Shifting and Care for the Uninsured," *Health Affairs* (Fall 1985), pp. 62–80.

6. See, for example, William Dudly, *The Clinton Health Care Plan: No Free Lunch* (Report of U.S. Economic Research, Goldman Sachs, Jan. 1994); and Martin Feldstein, "Clinton's Hidden Health Care Tax," *Wall Street Journal*, Nov. 10, 1993; and "The Health Plan's Financing Gap," *Wall Street Journal*, Sept. 9, 1993.

7. In a recent estimate of the costs of the Clinton plan, Lewin-VHI, Inc., use premium costs that are approximately 17 percent above the administration's for all four family categories but are about 16 percent below the level of the Hewitt premiums (after adjusting for inflation between 1993 and 1998).

8. It has proved exceedingly difficult to establish empirically the extent to which cash wages respond to changes in fringe benefits or other noncash forms of compensation. See the review in Jonathan Gruber and

Alan B. Krueger, "The Incidence of Mandated Employer-Provided Insurance: Lesson from Workers' Compensation Insurance," in David Bradford, ed., *Tax Policy and the Economy*, NBER, vol. 5 (Cambridge, Mass.: MIT Press). Their original research in this article suggests that more than 80 percent of mandated workers' compensation premiums were shifted to workers, which is a greater wage shift than typically has been estimated. Workers affected by this mandate, however, have significantly higher wages than workers who currently lack health insurance coverage.

9. For a review of the evidence, see Charles Brown, Curtis Gilroy, and Andrew Kohen, "The Effect of the Minimum Wage on Employment and Unemployment," *Journal of Economic Literature*, vol. 20 (June 1982).

10. David Card and Alan B. Krueger, *Minimum Wages and Employment: A Case Study of the Fast Food Industry in New Jersey and Pennsylvania* (Unpublished paper, March 1993); and Lawrence F. Katz and Alan B. Krueger, "The Effect of the Minimum Wage on the Fast Food Industry," *Industrial and Labor Relations Review*, vol. 46, no. 1 (October 1992).

11. Lowell J. Taylor and Taeil Kim, *The Employment Effect in Retail Trade of California's 1988 Minimum Wage Increase* (Unpublished paper, February 1993); David Card, "Do Minimum Wages Reduce Employment? A Case Study of California, 1987–1989; and David B. Neumark and William J. Wascher, "Employment Effects of Minimum and Sub-Minimum Wages: Panel Data on State Minimum Wage Laws," *Industrial and Labor Relations Review*, vol. 46, no. 1 (October 1992).

12. The authors of the two studies of fast food restaurants consider only short-run changes in employment within a fixed number of firms. Therefore, their results do not include the effect of the minimum on the rate of entry of new firms or on firm closing, which would be major factors affecting employment. Moreover, their analyses were confined entirely to restaurants belonging to three large national chains, which may be atypical in a number of ways. The results, therefore, may be limited.

13. Ronald G. Ehrenberg and Robert S. Smith, *Modern Labor Economics*, 4th ed. (New York: Harper Collins Publishers, Inc., 1992), pp. 115–35.

14. Daniel Hamermesh, *Labor Demand* (Princeton, N.J.: Princeton University Press, 1993), chap. 3.

15. Joseph E. Stiglitz, *Economics* (New York: W.W. Norton Company, 1993), table 5.1, p. 112.

16. We use different elasticity values across specific industries, constraining the sum of the individual industry impact to add to the aggregate value obtained using (-.3).

17. There are many other factors that would also influence an employer's premium costs in the transition from the current system to the

Clinton plan. For example, firms may provide benefits that are lower in cost because they are below the standard required by the plan and their costs would increase. Premiums under the current system are typically set using experience rating, which could produce higher or lower costs than the community rating required under the plan. These factors and many others could cause important differences. But they are difficult if not impossible to estimate with currently available data.

18. The large premium cost increase for this group in part arises because of a peculiar aspect of the Clinton subsidy scheme. High-wage workers in firms with enough low-wage workers, so that 7.9 percent of total payroll is less than total premium cost, will pay an amount 7.9 percent of their high-wage that in many cases will exceed the actual premium cost of their policy.

19. For additional discussion of these inefficiencies, see Henry J. Aaron, *Issues Every Plan to Reform Health Care Financing Must Confront* (Paper presented at the annual meetings of the American Economic Association, January 1994).

20. This example assumes that the firm is receiving a subsidy—that is, its average premium cost exceeds $24,000 x .079, or $1,896. If the cap amount exceeds the premium cost, then the insurance cost for the $15,000 worker would equal the premium cost (see discussion below). The same reasoning applies to the other examples in this paragraph.

21. See Alan B. Krueger, "Observations on Employment-based Government Mandates, with Particular Reference to Health Insurance" (Paper presented at the MIJCF conference "Labor Economics, Employment Policy and Job Creation," Washington, D.C., Nov. 1993).

About the Authors

JUNE E. O'NEILL is director of the Center for the Study of Business and Government and professor of economics and finance at Baruch College and the Graduate Center, City University of New York. Previously, she was director of the Office of Programs, Policy and Research at the U.S. Commission on Civil Rights. She has also directed a multidisciplinary research program (women and family policy) at the Urban Institute and has served as chief of the Human Resources Cost Estimates Unit of the Congressional Budget Office. Dr. O'Neill was a member of the senior staff of the President's Council of Economic Advisers specializing in issues related to the labor market, education, and income security programs. She is the author of numerous articles and books including her most recent article, "Income Discrimination and Income Differences," in *Race and Gender,* edited by Susan Feiner.

DAVE M. O'NEILL joined the Center for the Study of Business and Government in 1991 as a senior research associate, directing studies in health policy, labor economics, and education. He is currently conducting projects on the impact of rising costs of employer-based health insurance on changes in health insurance coverage during the 1980s, and on labor displacement effects of an employer health insurance mandate. Before joining the Center, Dr. O'Neill had extensive experience as an economist in both the academic and the policy sectors. He has taught at Pace University, the University of Pennsylvania, and Baruch College. Dr. O'Neill worked in Washington, D.C., senior level positions in economic policy analysis at both private research institutes and government agencies. He is the author of numerous works, including *The Impact of a Health Insurance Mandate on Labor Costs and Employment* (co-written with June O'Neill).

AEI Studies in Health Policy

Special Studies in Health Reform

ECONOMIC EFFECTS OF HEALTH REFORM
C. Eugene Steuerle

THE EMPLOYMENT AND DISTRIBUTIONAL EFFECTS OF MANDATED BENEFITS
June E. O'Neill and Dave M. O'Neill

GLOBAL BUDGETS VS. COMPETITIVE COST CONTROL STRATEGIES
Patricia M. Danzon

IS COMMUNITY RATING ESSENTIAL TO MANAGED COMPETITION?
Mark A. Hall

REMAKING HEALTH ALLIANCES
Clark C. Havighurst

UNHEALTHY ALLIANCES: BUREAUCRATS, INTEREST GROUPS, AND
POLITICIANS IN HEALTH REFORM
Henry N. Butler

Other AEI Books on Health Policy

HEALTH POLICY REFORM: COMPETITION AND CONTROLS
Edited by Robert B. Helms

AMERICAN HEALTH POLICY: CRITICAL ISSUES FOR REFORM
Edited by Robert B. Helms

HEALTH CARE POLICY AND POLITICS: LESSONS FROM FOUR COUNTRIES
Edited by Robert B. Helms

RESPONSIBLE NATIONAL HEALTH INSURANCE
Mark V. Pauly, Patricia Danzon, Paul J. Feldstein, and John Hoff

REGULATING DOCTORS' FEES: COMPETITION, BENEFITS,
AND CONTROLS UNDER MEDICARE
Edited by H. E. Frech III

www.ingramcontent.com/pod-product-compliance
Lightning Source LLC
Jackson TN
JSHW011944131224
75386JS00041B/1555

* 9 7 8 0 8 4 4 7 7 0 2 1 5 *